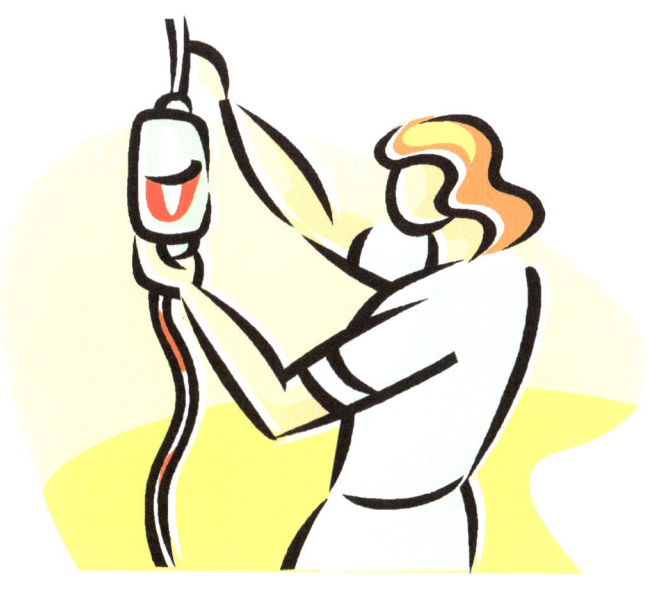

Medical/Surgical Nursing Skills Made Simple

Understanding the Importance behind the

Skill

By: Maureen Kroning MSN RN

<u>Dedication</u>

This book is dedicated to all of the caring and hardworking nurses who provide patients, families and communities with competent and safe nursing care each and every day.

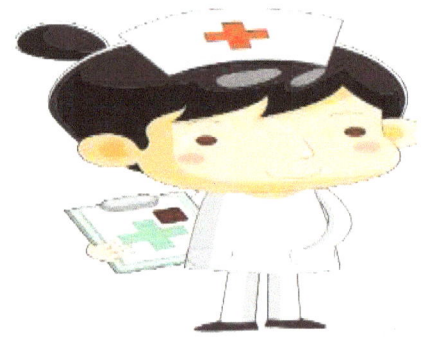

Table of Contents

Topics   **Page #**

Oxygen Therapy

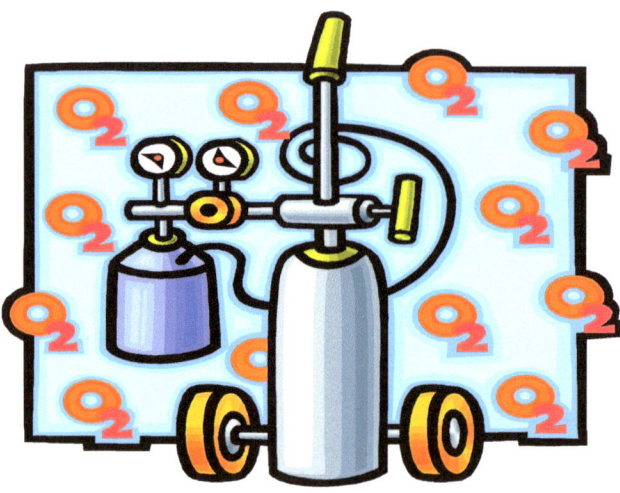

1. What equipment is needed when placing a patient on O2 therapy?

   _____

2. Do you need a doctor's order to administer oxygen to a patient?

   _____

3. Can the nurse delegate the application of oxygen administration to nursing assistive personnel?

   _____

4. What assessments are necessary prior to oxygen administration?

   _____

5. What position should the bed be in, if not contraindicated, to provide for optimal lung expansion and help to ease respiratory effort?

   _____

6. What percentage of FiO2 can be delivered by nasal cannula?

   _____

7. What percentage of FiO2 is 1/L min delivered by nasal cannula?

_____

8. What percentage of FiO2 is 2/L min delivered by nasal cannula?

_____

9. What percentage of FiO2 is 3/L min delivered by nasal cannula?

_____

10. What percentage of FiO2 is 4/L min delivered by nasal cannula?

_____

11. What percentage of FiO2 is 5/L min delivered by nasal cannula?

_____

12. What percentage of FiO2 is 6/L min delivered by nasal cannula?

_____

13. What are the advantages of oxygen delivery by nasal cannula?

_____

14. What are the disadvantages of using nasal cannula for oxygen administration?

_____

15. What percentage of FiO2 can be delivered by a simple face mask?

_____

16. What percentage of FiO2 is 5-6L/min delivered by a simple face mask?

_____

17. What percentage of FiO2 is 6-7L/min delivered by a simple face mask?

_____

18. What percentage of FiO2 is 7-8L /min delivered by a simple face mask?

_____

19. What is an advantage of using a simple face mask to administer oxygen to a patient?

_____

20. What are the disadvantages of administering oxygen by a simple face mask?

_____

21. What percentage of FiO2 can be delivered by a Venturi mask?

_____

22. What percentage of FiO2 is 4/L min delivered by a Venturi mask?

_____

23. What percentage of FiO2 is 8/L min delivered by a Venturi mask?

_____

24. What percentage of FiO2 is 12/L min delivered by a Venturi mask?

_____

25. What are the advantages of delivering oxygen by a Venturi mask?

_____

26. What are the disadvantages of delivering oxygen through a Venturi mask?

_____

27. When using a partial non breather to deliver oxygen how should the bag attached remain?

_____

28. What percentage of FiO2 can be delivered by a partial non breather mask?

_____

29. What percentage of FiO2 is 6L/min delivered by a partial non breather mask?

_____

30. What percentage of FiO2 is 7L/min delivered by a partial non breather mask?

_____

31. What percentage of FiO2 is 8L/min delivered by a partial non breather mask?

_____

32. What percentage of FiO2 is 9L/min delivered by a partial non breather mask?

_____

33. What percentage of FiO2 is 10L/min delivered by a partial non breather mask?

_____

34. What are the advantages of delivering oxygen by a partial non breather mask?

_____

35. What are the disadvantages of delivering oxygen by a partial non breather mask?

_____

36. How much FiO2 can be delivered by a non breather mask?

_____

37. What are the advantages of delivering oxygen by a non breather face mask?

_____

38. What are the disadvantages of delivering oxygen by a non breather mask?

_____

39. How much FiO2 can be delivered by a face tent?

_____

40. What is the advantage of delivering oxygen by a face tent?

_____

41. What are the disadvantages of delivering oxygen by a face tent?

_____

42. How much FiO2 can be delivered by an oxygen hood?

_____

43. What are the advantages of delivering oxygen by an oxygen hood?

_____

44. What are the disadvantages of delivering oxygen by an oxygen hood?

_____

45. What percentage of FiO2 can be delivered by an oxygen tent?

_____

46. What are the advantages of delivering oxygen by an oxygen tent?

_____

47. What are the disadvantages of delivering oxygen by an oxygen tent?

_____

Using an Incentive Spirometer

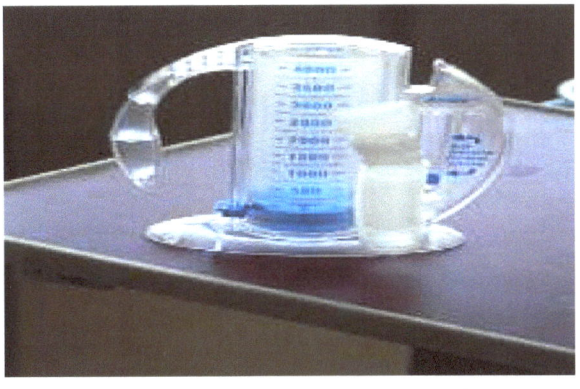

1. What is an incentive spirometer used for?

   _____

2. When is it common for the nurse to teach and encourage a patient about the benefits of

   using an incentive spirometer?

   _____

3. Can the nurse delegate, to nursing assistive personnel, assisting patients with the use of

   an incentive spirometer?

   _____

4. What post operative complication can an incentive spirometer help prevent?

   _____

5. Along with the use of an incentive spirometer, what other pulmonary hygiene techniques

   can benefit patients post operatively?

   _____

6. What are the two types of incentive spirometer devices that are frequently used in the

   healthcare setting?

   _____

7. Which of the two incentive spirometer devices has one or two plastic chambers that contain free moveable colored balls?

_____

8. What is the advantage of the flow-oriented incentive spirometer device?

_____

9. Which of the two incentive spirometer devices has a bellow that the patient inhales slowly to rise?

_____

10. What is the advantage of a volume-oriented incentive spirometer device?

_____

.

Suctioning

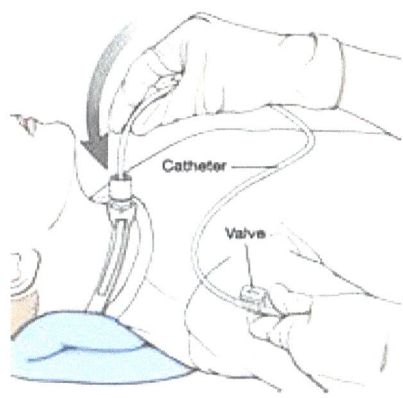

1. What equipment is necessary to suction a patient?

_____

2. What type of suction catheter would be used for oropharyngeal suctioning?

_____

3. Can oropharyngeal suctioning be delegated to unlicensed personnel?

_____

4. What should the nurse avoid when performing oropharyngeal suctioning?

_____

5. What assessment should the nurse do prior to suctioning?

_____

6. What findings should the nurse chart after suctioning a patient?

_____

7. Where does oropharyngeal suctioning remove secretions from?

_____

8. Where does tracheal suctioning remove secretions from?

_____

9. What can occur if secretions are not removed from a patient's airway?

    _____

10. What are the risks associated with suctioning?

    _____

11. In order to suction out secretions what type of pressure is placed on the catheter as it is drawn out of the patient's airway?

    _____

12. What are two types of artificial airway?

    _____

13. Which of the two artificial airways is considered to be temporary?

    _____

14. Which of the artificial airways can be placed permanently?

    _____

15. Can suctioning of a nasotracheal and a new artificial airway be delegated to nursing assistive personnel?

    _____

16. When can suctioning a patient via tracheostomy be delegated to unlicensed personnel?

    _____

17. What are the contraindications to nasotracheal suctioning?

    _____

18. During what phase of respirations does the nurse put in the suction catheter?

    _____

19. Why does the nurse avoid placing a suction catheter in while a patient is swallowing?

_____

20. When should the nurse apply suction to the suction caterer?

_____

21. What can the patient do, if possible, to help advance the suction catheter if it has difficulty passing?

_____

22. In what order, if possible, should the nurse perform nasal, tracheal and pharyngeal suctioning?

_____

23. What should the nurse monitor the patient for when performing suctioning?

_____

24. In what patients is suctioning limited to approximately two times per suction procedure?

_____

25. What should the nurse do if the patient shows signs of respiratory distress during suctioning?

_____

Care of a Tracheostomy

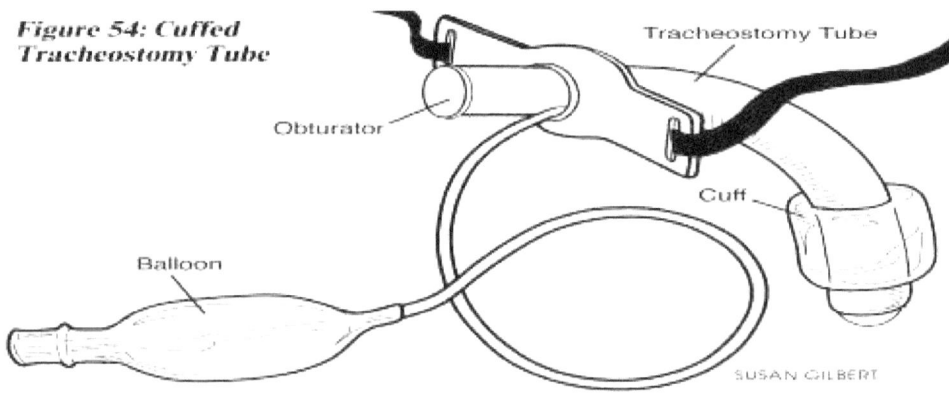

Figure 54: Cuffed Tracheostomy Tube

Tracheostomy Tube

Obturator

Cuff

Balloon

SUSAN GILBERT

1. What is a tracheostomy?

   _____

2. What equipment is needed to perform tracheostomy care?

   _____

3. When the patient has a tracheostomy what equipment should be taped above the

   patient's bed or visible at the bedside?

   _____

4. What are signs to indicate that tracheostomy care is necessary?

   _____

5. When performing tracheostomy care what should the nurse assess the stoma for?

   _____

6. What does the nurse need to record after tracheostomy care is completed?

   _____

Chest tube care

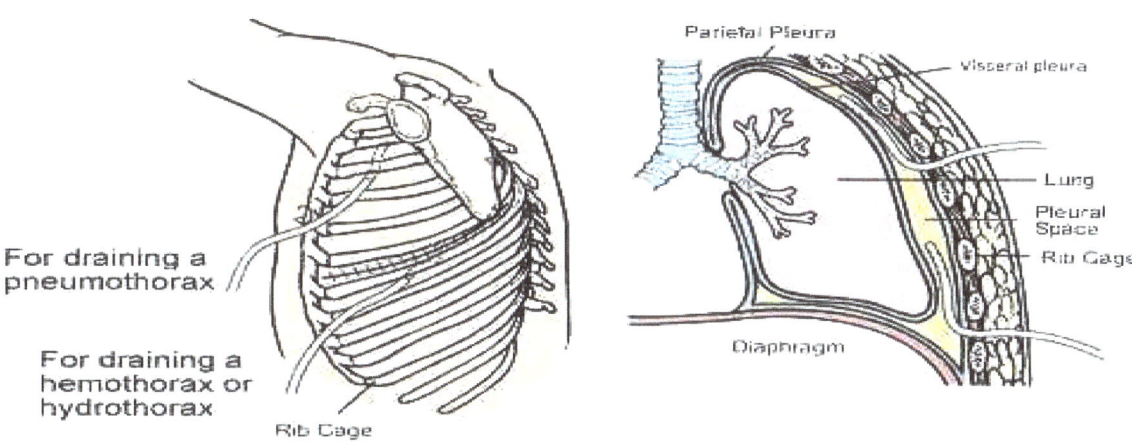

1. What can cause a patient to require a chest tube?

   _____

2. What can cause the collapse of lung tissue?

   _____

3. Where is the chest tube inserted?

   _____

4. Can the placement of the chest tube in the thorax tell us what is going to be removed

   from the pleural space?

   _____

5. The placement of a chest tube in apical and anterior placement is generally used to

   remove what?

   _____

6. The placement of a chest tube low (fifth/sixth intercostal space) posterior or lateral is generally used to remove what?

_____

7. The placement of a mediastinal chest tube is generally used to remove what?

_____

8. After what type of surgery would the nurse expect to see a mediastinal chest tube in a patient?

_____

9. What type of system is attached to the chest tube of a patient in order to remove air, fluid or blood?

_____

10. What can the chest tube remove from the pleural space?

_____

11. What type of pressure in the intrapleural space causes the lung to collapse?

_____

12. What is an increase in pleural fluid called?

_____

13. What are the two classifications of pleural effusion?

_____

14. What types of conditions can lead to a transudate effusion?

_____

15. What types of conditions can lead to an exudate effusion?

_____

16. What is the term used when the lung collapses?

_____

17. What is the type of pnemothorax when a patient experiences chest trauma?

_____

18. What is the type of pnemothorax a patient can develop as a result of the rupturing of a small bleb on the lung or from the insertion of a subclavian intravenous line?

_____

19. What is the type of pnemothorax a patient can develop as a result of a disease process such as emphysema?

_____

20. What is the type of pnemothorax a patient can develop as a result of a rupture in the pleura?

_____

21. What untoward side effect can occur with a tension pneumothorax that is left untreated?

_____

22. What symptoms may occur if the patient displays untoward side effects as a result of an untreated tension pneumothorax?

_____

23. What is the type of pneumothorax a patient can develop as a result of the accumulation of blood and fluid in the pleural cavity?

_____

IV Therapy

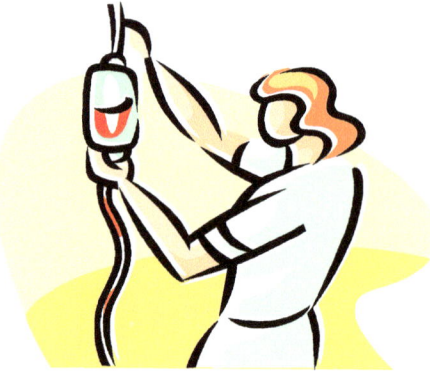

1. What does IV stand for?

   _____

2. What can be given IV to patients?

   _____

3. What are the six patient rights to be followed during IV treatment?

   _____

4. What are three types of IV solutions?

   _____

5. Which solution has the same osmolarity of blood?

   _____

6. What are examples of isotonic IVsolutions?

   _____

7. What IV solutions have an osmolarity that is less than that the body fluids?

   _____

8. What is an example of a hypotonic IV solution?

9. What IV solutions have an osmolarity that is greater than that of the body fluids?

_____

10. What are examples of hypertonic IV solutions?

_____

11. What IV solution is likely to be ordered for a patient with prolonged vomiting?

_____

12. Which of the three IV solutions would most likely cause pulmonary edema if the IV is not carefully monitored?

_____

13. What size gauge catheter would likely be inserted in an adult patient for an IV infusion?

_____

14. What size gauge catheter would likely be inserted in a pediatric patient for an IV infusion?

_____

15. What safety measures help prevent needle stick injuries?

_____

16. What is the recommended time that the IV catheter site is rotated and the IV tubing changed?

_____

17. Why are guidelines and recommendations in place to change the IV catheter and tubing?

_____

18. What are three complications associated with an IV?

_____

19. What symptoms indicate an IV site infection?

_____

20. What symptoms indicate an IV site infiltration?

_____

21. What are symptoms associated with an IV site phlebitis?

_____

22. What should the nurse do if infection, infiltration or phlebitis occurs?

_____

23. What is important to do to the patient's skin prior to inserting an IV catheter?

_____

24. What types of IV catheters are most often used for short term use?

_____

25. What types of IV catheters are most often used for long term use?

_____

26. What are examples of central venous access devices (CVAD)?

_____

27. What are other advantages to using a CVAD other than for long term use?

_____

28. What patient assessment findings are important for the nurse to assess for prior to IV administration?

_____

29. What does the nurse need to do in the event he/she sustains a needle stick injury?

_____

30. What is the name of the organization that requires needle-stick reporting?

_____

31. Can the nurse delegate the insertion of a peripheral IV line to nursing assistive personnel?

_____

Administering Blood Transfusions

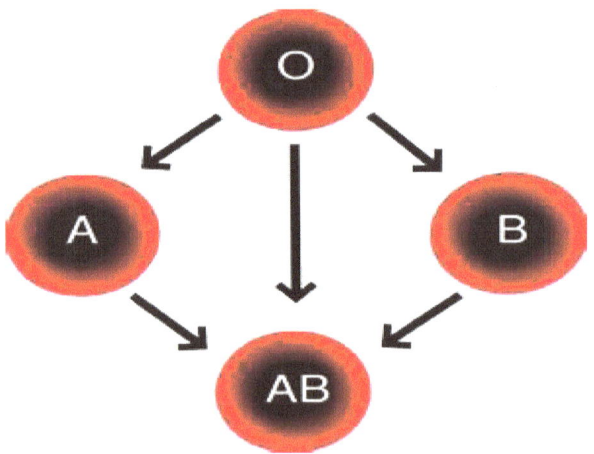

1. Does the nurse need a healthcare providers order to administer blood to a patient?

   _____

2. Is consent required to administer blood to a patient?

   _____

3. What patient test needs to be completed before administering blood?

   _____

4. What does a type and cross test tell us about the patient?

   _____

5. What is the ideal temperature to infuse blood on a patient?

   _____

6. What can the administration of cold blood cause?

   _____

7. Can the nurse delegate the administration of blood to nursing assistive personnel?

   _____

8. What blood component does not run the risk of transmitting HIV/ HBV when providing a transfusion?

_____

9. What blood product is used to increase red blood cells and plasma volume?

_____

10. What blood product is commonly used to raise Hgb/Hct levels?

_____

11. What blood product is commonly administered to patients with thrombocytopenia?

_____

12. What vital signs are taken prior to the administration of a blood transfusion?

_____

13. What adverse reactions does the nurse assesses for when administering a blood transfusion?

_____

14. What can the presence of a fever indicate during a blood transfusion?

_____

15. What can the presence of tachycardia, tacypnea and dyspnea indicate during a blood transfusion?

_____

16. What can the presence of hives, skin rash and or flushing indicate during a blood transfusion?

_____

17. Besides an allergic reaction, what can the presence of flushing indicate during a blood transfusion?

_____

18. What can the presence of nausea and or vomiting indicate during a blood transfusion?

_____

19. What can the presence of diarrhea indicate during a blood transfusion?

_____

20. What can the presence of hypotension indicate during a blood transfusion?

_____

21. What can the presence of crackles in the base of the lungs indicate during a blood transfusion?

_____

22. If the nurse notices any adverse reactions while administering a blood transfusion, he/she should do what?

_____

23. What does the nurse need to document in the patient's chart when administering a blood transfusion?

_____

Naso-Gastric and Naso-Enteric Tube Feeding Care

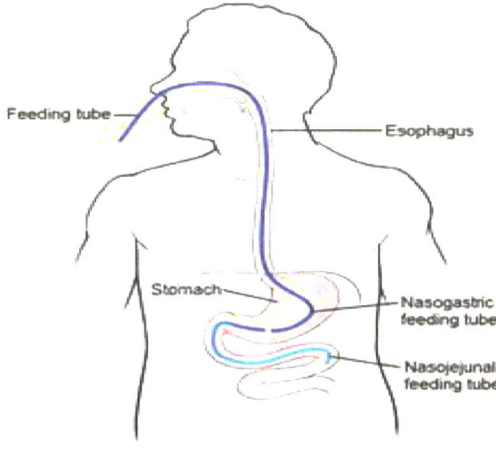

1. What is the abbreviated term for a naso gastric tube?

    _____

2. What are naso gastric tubes be used for?

    _____

3. What patients should not have the placement of an NG tube?

    _____

4. Does the insertion of a feeding tube require a healthcare provider's order?

    _____

5. Can the nurse delegate verification of NG tube placement to nursing assistive

    personnel?

    _____

6. Can the nurse delegate the administration of a NG tube feeding to nursing assistive

    personnel?

    _____

7. What is considered a major risk factor when administering NG tube feedings?

_____

8. Where on the patient can the nurse insert a small bore NG feeding tube?

_____

9. How does the nurse measure the NG tube to ensure that it reaches the patients

   stomach?

_____

10. What is the recommended patient positioning for NG tube insertion?

_____

11. What is the recommended way to initially verify if a NG tube is placed properly?

_____

12. After the initial verification of a NG tube placement, how often should the nurse

    assess verification by another method such as pH testing prior to using the NG tube

    for feedings?

_____

13. When inserting a NG tube in a patient, what symptoms would cause the nurse to stop

    advancing the tube?

_____

14. What factors can increase the patient's risk for dislodging the NG tube and

    aspirating?

_____

15. If a patient cannot tolerate a small bore feeding tube or requires long term tube feedings, what type of feeding tube may be inserted directly into the stomach?

_____

16. Who inserts a gastrostomy feeding tube?

_____

17. What is the feeding tube that is inserted in the jejunum called?

_____

18. Can the nurse delegate care of a gastrostomy or jejunostomy tube to nursing assistive personnel?

_____

19. How long generally can the formula in an open system tube feeding hang up for?

_____

20. How long generally can the formula in an closed system tube feeding hang up for?

_____

Care of Urinary Catheters

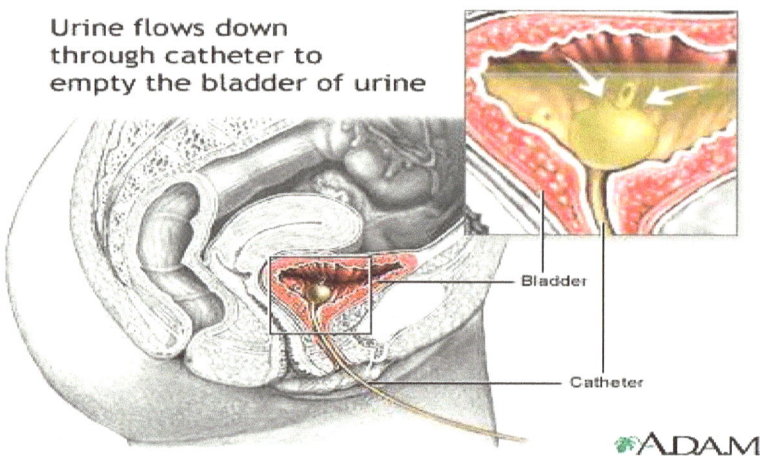

Urine flows down through catheter to empty the bladder of urine

Bladder

Catheter

ADAM.

1. Does the nurse need an order to insert a urinary catheter?

_____

2. Can insertion of a straight or indwelling catheter be delegated to nursing assistive

   personnel?

_____

3. Can the task of routine urinary catheter care and the removal of a urinary catheter be

   delegated to nursing assistive personnel?

_____

4. What should the nurse document after inserting a urinary catheter?

_____

5. When inserting a urinary catheter where does the nurse insert the catheter?

_____

6. After inserting the urinary catheter into the patient's urethra where is it advanced to?

_____

7. When inserting a urinary catheter in a female patient and there is no evidence of urine output and the possibility that the catheter is in the vagina what can the nurse do to assist placing a new catheter into the urethra?

_____

8. When inserting a urinary catheter in a male patient and there is noted resistance what can the nurse instruct the patient to do to help him relax?

_____

9. What should the nurse do when inserting a urinary catheter in a male patient and there's noted resistance even after the patient does relaxation techniques?

_____

10. What is the name used to describe the catheter that is used to intermittently remove urine from the bladder, take a sterile urine sample or check for residual urine in the patient's bladder?

_____

11. What is the name used to describe the catheter that is used for short or long term use and is attached to a closed drainage system?

_____

12. What is the separate lumen that is attached to the foley used for?

_____

13. What should the nurse do if when inflating the balloon on the foley catheter causes the patient to experience pain?

_____

14. What are reasons that a foley or an indwelling catheter may be inserted?

_____

15. What assessment findings should the nurse note in reference to collecting urine?

_____

16. What is the height level that a patient's urine collection container is placed at?

_____

17. What size catheter can cause damage to the urethra, bladder neck and can cause bladder

spasms when inserted?

_____

18. What catheter care is important for the nurse to do in order to prevent bacterial growth

around the urinary catheter?

_____

19. When removing an indwelling urinary catheter, the nurse must do what to the inflation

valve?

_____

20. If the nurse removes the sterile water from the inflation valve and feels resistance while

removing the indwelling catheter the nurse should do what?

_____

Answers

Oxygen Therapy

1. The equipment needed when placing a patient on O2 therapy is an oxygen flow meter, the type of oxygen administration device and sterile water if the device requires humidification.

2. Yes, administering oxygen to a patient requires specific orders by the doctor or designated health care provider. The order should include the date, time, physician name and signature, medical record number and the type and amount of oxygen delivery ordered.

3. Yes, the nurse can delegate the task of applying a nasal cannula and most other types of mask oxygen delivery systems. However the nurse may not delegate the task of applying oxygen via a tracheostomy collar.

4. Prior to oxygen administration it is necessary to assess the patient's: respiratory status, signs and symptoms associated with difficulty breathing, vital signs, Hgb level and oxygen saturation level.

5. The head of the bed should be placed in a mid to high fowlers position to ease respiratory effort and expand the patient's lung.

6. 1-6/L min and 24-44% of FiO2 can be delivered by nasal cannula.

7. 1L/ min is equivalent to 24% of FiO2 delivery by nasal cannula.

8. 2L/ min is equivalent to 28% of FiO2 delivery by nasal cannula.

9. 3L/ min is equivalent to 32% of FiO2 delivery by nasal cannula.

10. 4L/ min is equivalent to 36% of FiO2 delivery by nasal cannula.

11. 5L/ min is equivalent to 40% of FiO2 delivery by nasal cannula.

12. 6L/ min is equivalent to 44% of FiO2 delivery by nasal cannula.

13. The advantages of administering oxygen via a nasal cannula are: it is considered safe, simple, easily tolerated, inexpensive, can deliver low oxygen concentrations and the patient can eat and speak while the nasal cannula is in place.

14. The disadvantages of using nasal cannula for oxygen administration are: can not be used with nasal obstruction, it is drying to the mucus membranes, can dislodge easily, may cause skin irritation or breakdown and the exact amount of oxygen delivered is dependent on the patient's breathing pattern.

15. A simple face mask can deliver 5 to greater than 8L/min and 40-60% of FiO2.

16. 5-6L/min is equivalent to 40% of FiO2 delivery by a simple face mask.

17. 6-7L/min is equivalent to 50% of FiO2 delivery by a simple face mask.

18. 7-8L/min is equivalent to 60% of FiO2 delivery by a simple face mask.

19. The advantage of using a simple face mask to deliver oxygen to a patient is that a simple face mask can provide humidification when the oxygen is delivered.

20. The disadvantages of delivering oxygen by a simple face mask are: the exact oxygen amount can be difficult to achieve, it requires a high level of oxygen in order to prevent the patient from breathing in CO2 and the patient will breath in room air through the side holes.

21. 4-12/L min and 24-60% of FiO2 can be delivered by a venturi mask.

22. 4L/ min is equivalent to 24-28% of FiO2 delivered by a venturi mask.

23. 8L/ min is equivalent to 35-40% of FiO2 delivered by a venturi mask.

24. 12L/ min is equivalent to 50-60% of FiO2 delivered by a venturi mask.

25. The advantages of delivering oxygen by a venturi mask are: the amount of oxygen delivery can be controlled, can deliver between 24-60% oxygen concentration, does not dry the mucus membranes and provides humidification.

26. The disadvantages of delivering oxygen through a Venturi mask are: it is considered to be hot, confining, the humidification can irritate the skin, if the mask does not fit right the amount of oxygen can be decreased and it interferes with both eating and talking.

27. The bag attached to a partial non breather oxygen delivery system needs to remain partially inflated at all times.

28. A partial non breather mask can deliver 6-10L/min and 60-95% of FiO2.

29. 6L/min is equivalent to 60% of FiO2 delivered by a partial non breather mask.

30. 7L/min is equivalent to 70% of FiO2 delivered by a partial non breather mask.

31. 8L/min is equivalent to 80% of FiO2 delivered by a partial non breather mask.

32. 9L/min is equivalent to 90% of FiO2 delivered by a partial non breather mask.

33. 10L/min is equivalent to 95% of FiO2 delivered by a partial non breather mask.

34. The advantages of delivering oxygen by a partial non breather mask are: it can deliver increased amounts of oxygen, is easily humidified and does not dry the mucus membranes.

35. The disadvantages of delivering oxygen by a partial non breather mask are: there is expiratory and inspiratory air mix, it can be hot, confining, irritate skin and it can interfere with eating and talking.

36. A non breather mask can deliver 6-15L/min and 60-100% of FiO2.

37. The advantages of delivering oxygen by a non breather face mask are: the exhaled air does not mix with inhaled air; it can deliver the highest possible oxygen and does not dry the mucus membranes.

38. The disadvantage of delivering oxygen by a non breather masks are: it needs to have a tight seal, it can be difficult to maintain, uncomfortable, can irritate the skin and the bag has to stay inflated.

39. A face tent can deliver 8-12L/min and 28-100% of FiO2.

40. The advantage of delivering oxygen by a face tent is that it is a good alternative method of delivering oxygen while providing high humidity.

41. The disadvantages of delivering oxygen by a face tent are: it is difficult to keep in place and the oxygen level cannot be controlled.

42. An oxygen hood can deliver 5-12L/min and 28-85% of FiO2.

43. The advantages of delivering oxygen by an oxygen hood are: it provides warmed humidified oxygen and it is a good method of delivering oxygen for pediatric patients.

44. The disadvantage of delivering oxygen by a oxygen hood is that having the flow rate set at a level of less than 5L/min can result in CO2 narcosis.

45. An oxygen tent can deliver 10-15L/min and up to 50% of FiO2.

46. The advantages of delivering oxygen by a oxygen tent are: it provides both humidified and cool temperature and a good source for delivering oxygen for pediatric patients.

47. The disadvantages of delivering oxygen by a oxygen tent are: it can be isolating for a child and when the tent is opened the oxygen and humidity level will change.

Incentive Spirometer

1. Incentive spirometry is used to encourage and assist patients to take deep breaths.

2. It is common to teach and encourage patients how to use incentive spirometry prior to and after: abdominal, cardiac, thoracic and orthopedic surgeries, patients at risk for developing respiratory complications from an illness or a surgical procedure or as a result of bed rest.

3. Yes, the nurse can delegate to nursing assistive personnel assisting patients with the use of incentive spirometry.

4. The use of the incentive spirometry can help prevent pulmonary atelectasis or postoperative pneumonia.

5. The use of chest physical therapy, coughing and deep breathing exercises and intermittent positive pressure can also be used in conjuncture with the use of the incentive spirometry to help prevent postoperative pulmonary complications.

6. The two types of incentive spirometry devices that are frequently used in the health care setting are flow- oriented and volume- oriented devices.

7. The flow- oriented incentive spirometry device has one or tows plastic chambers that contain freely moveable colored balls.

8. The advantage of the flow-oriented incentive spirometry device is that the patient is encouraged to take slow deep breaths.

9. The volume-oriented incentive spirometry devices has a bellow that patient inhales slowly to rise.

10. The advantage of the volume-oriented incentive spirometry device is that the patient can both accomplish and measure their inspiratory volume.

Suctioning

1. The equipment that is needed to suction a patient includes the proper size catheter for either nasal of oral suctioning, sterile and clean gloves, wall or portable suction machine, mask, goggles or face shield if risk of contamination or isolation precautions require them, connecting tubing, water-soluble lubricant, sterile container with sterile saline solution, a pulse oxcimeter and a stethoscope.

2. A Yankauer suction catheter is used for oropharyngeal suctioning.

3. Yes, oropharyngeal suctioning can be delegated to unlicensed personnel unless the patient is in the postoperative phase after having any oral or neck surgery.

4. The nurse needs to avoid excessive pressure, any mouth sutures, sensitive tissue areas and any tubes that may be present and avoid the patient gag reflex when performing oropharyngeal suctioning.

5. The nurse should assess the patients understanding of suctioning and its purpose, the oxygen saturation of the patient any signs of altered respiratory status and risk factors such as airway obstruction, impaired cough, gag, swallowing and the patient's level of consciousness.

6. The nurse should record the color, odor, consistency, amount and the frequency of the suctioning required.

7. Oropharangeal suctioning removes secretions from the mouth and the back of the throat.

8. Tracheal suctioning can remove secretions from both the upper and lower airway.

9. A patient can develop an infection, aspiration, pneumonia or respiratory failure if secretions are not removed from the airways.

10. The risks associated with suctioning patients include hypoxemia, cardiac spasms, dysrhythmias, laryngeal spasms, bradycardia, and trauma and bleeding.

11. Negative pressure must be placed on the catheter as it is drawn out of the patient's airway in order to suction out secretions.

12. The two types of artificial airways include: endotracheal tube and tracheostomy tube.

13. The endotracheal tube is considered to be temporary.

14. The tracheostomy tube can be placed permanently.

15. No, suctioning of a nasotracheal and a new artificial airway cannot be delegated to nursing assistive personnel.

16. Suctioning a patient through a tracheostomy site can be delegated to unliscnesed personnel if the tracheostomy is stable and is not newly placed.

17. Contraindications to nasotracheal suctioning include: facial or neck trauma/surgery, bleeding, epiglottitis or croup, laryngospasm, irritable airway and gastric surgery with high anastomosis.

18. The suction catheter is placed into the patient's airway during inspiration.

19. The nurse should avoid placing a suction catheter in while a patient is swallowing to prevent the catheter from entering into the esophagus.

20. The nurse applies suction to the suction catheter while removing it from the patient's airway.

21. The patient can cough or say "ahh" if they are able to assist and the suction catheter is difficult to pass in to the airway.

22. The nurse should first suction the nasal and tracheal airways before suctioning the pharyngeal airway.

23. The nurse should monitor the patient's vital signs, oxygen saturation and level of comfort during suctioning.

24. Patients with increased intracranial pressure should receive a limit to only two times of suctioning during each suctioning procedure.

25. The nurse or nursing assistive personnel should immediately withdraw the suction caterer and provide supplemental oxygen if needed as well as notify the healthcare provider of the incident.

Care of a Tracheostomy

1. A tracheostomy is the surgical procedure of an artificial airway into the trachea.

2. The supplies needed to complete tracheostomy care include: a towel, suction supplies, tracheostomy care kit, two pairs of clean gloves and a mask, goggles and face shield.

3. A replacement tracheostomy with the correct size and manufacturer needs to be at the patient's bedside.

4. Signs that the nurse may see to indicate that tracheostomy care is necessary include: copious secretions, damp tracheostomy ties and or dressing, decreased air flow and any signs of obstruction.

5. The stoma should be assessed for any sign of infection, bleeding, and skin breakdown.

6. The nurse needs to record the time, date, tracheostomy tube type and size, description of the care provided, assessment findings and patient's tolerance to the tracheostomy care.

Chest tube care

1. Certain disease processes, traumatic injuries and surgical procedures could cause the need for a chest tube to be inserted.

2. The leakage of air, blood or fluid into the intrapleural space can cause the lung to collapse.

3. The chest tube is inserted in the thorax.

4. Yes, the placement of the chest tube can generally tell us what if it is air, fluid or blood.

5. The placement of a chest tube in apical (second/third intercostal space) and anterior placement is generally used to remove air.

6. The placement of a chest tube low (fifth/sixth intercoastal space) posterior or lateral is generally used to remove fluid.

7. The placement of a medialstinal chest tube is generally used to remove blood or fluid.

8. After open heart surgery the nurse would expect to see a mediastinal chest tube in a patient.

9. A closed chest drainage system with or without suction is attached to the chest tube of a patient in order to remove air, fluid or blood.

10. The chest tube removes air, blood or fluid form the pleural space.

11. Positive pressure in the intrapleural space causes the lung to collapse.

12. An increase in pleural fluid is called pleural effusion.

13. The two classifications of a pleural effusion are transudate or exudate effusion.

14. Congestive heart failure, hepatic disease or nephritic syndromes are conditions can lead to a transudate effusion.

15. Cancer, infection, pancreatitis, connective tissue diseases or collagen vascular diseases can lead to an exudate effusion.

16. A pneumothorax is the term used when the lung collapses.

17. The type of pnemothorax a patient experiences with chest trauma is called a traumatic pnemothorax.

18. The type of pnemothorax a patient can develop as a result of the rupturing of a small bleb on the lung or from the insertion of a subcalvian intravenous line is called a spontaneous or primary pneumothorax.

19. The type of pnemothorax a patient can develop as a result of a disease process such as emphysema is called a secondary pneumothorax.

20. The type of pnemothorax a patient can develop as a result of a rupture in the pleura is called a tension pnumothorax.

21. The lung on the other side can collapse, a mediastinum shift and venous return and cardiac output can decrease if a tension pneumothorax is left untreated.

22. The symptoms that may occur if the patient displays untoward side effects as a result of an untreated tension pneumothorax include: sudden complaint of chest pain, a fall in the blood pressure, tachycardia and possible cardiac arrest.

23. The type of pnemothorax a patient can develop as a result of the accumulation of blood and fluid in the pleural cavity is called a hemothorax.

IV Therapy

1. IV stands for intravenous.

2. Fluids, blood products, electrolytes, medications, nutritional supplemental feedings can be given IV to patients.

3. The six patient rights to be followed during IV therapy include the: right patient, right route, right medication/solution, right dose, right date & time and the right documentation.

4. The three types of IV solutions include: isotonic, hypotonic and hypertonic.

5. Isotonic solutions have the same osmolartiy of blood.

6. Examples of isotonic IV solutions include: 0.9%NS and Lactated Ringers (LR).

7. Hypotonic solutions have an osmolarity that is less than that of the body fluids.

8. An example of a hypotonic IV solutions is 0.45%NS.

9. Hypertonic solutions have an osmolarity that is greater than that of the body fluids.

10. Examples of hypertonic IV solutions include: D51/2NS and D5NS.

11. An isotonic IV solution is likely to be ordered for a patient with prolonged vomiting.

12. A hypertonic IV solution can cause pulmonary edema by drawing water into the vascular space.

13. A 18-24 gauge catheter would likely be inserted in an adult patient for an IV infusion.

14. A 22-24 gauge catheter would likely be inserted in a pediatric patient for an IV infusion.

15. The use of needless safety system helps prevent needle stick injuries.

16. Every 72 hours is the recommended time that the IV catheter and IV tubing should be changed.

17. There are guidelines and recommendations in place to rotate the IV catheter site and change IV tubing to prevent complications associated with IV therapy.

18. Infection, infiltration and phlebitis are three complications associated with IV therapy.

19. Inflammation, pain, pruritis and temperature are symptoms associated with an IV site infection.

20. Inflammation, skin blanching, coolness, damp or wet dressing and the infusion has slowed or has stopped infusing are symptoms associated with an IV site infiltration.

21. Redness, pain or burning along the length of the vein, edema and the vein being hard or cordlike are symptoms associated with IVphlebitis.

22. The nurse should stop the IV infusion, call the medical provider and remove the IV catheter if infection, infiltration or phlebitis occurs.

23. Cleansing the patient's skin with an antiseptic solution is important for the nurse to do prior to inserting an IV catheter.

24. Peripherally inserted IV catheters are most often used for short term use.

25 Central venous access devices (CVAD) are most often used for long term use.

26. Non tunneled and tunneled catheters, peripherally inserted central catheters (PICC) and implanted ports are examples of central venous access devices.

27. Giving medications and solutions that can be irritating to the veins are other advantages to using a CVAD.

28. It is important for the nurse to assess the patient's: vital signs, body weight, skin turgor, neck veins, behavioral changes, capillary refill, elimination status and any signs of edema, anorexia, nausea and or vomiting.

29. The nurse needs to contact the floor manager, nursing supervisor, fill out an incident report and follow the healthcare protocol that is required by the healthcare facility.

30. Occupational Safety and Health Administration (OSHA) requires healthcare facilities to report all needle-sticks.

31. No, the nurse cannot delegate to nursing assistive personnel the insertion of a peripheral IV line.

Administering Blood Transfusions

1. Yes, the nurse needs a healthcare providers order to administer blood to a patient.

2. Yes, consent is required to administer blood to a patient.

3. Typing and compatibility screening often called a type and cross test, is completed on the patient before ordering the blood.

4. The type and cross test tells us the patient's blood type and the compatibility of the donors antibodies.

5. Room temperature is the ideal temperature to infuse blood on a patient.

6. Administering cold blood to a patient can cause dysrhythmias and a decrease in the patient core body temperature.

7. No, the nurse cannot delegate the administration of blood to nursing assistive personnel.

8. Colloid components do not run the risk of transmitting HIV/ HBV infection.

9. Whole blood is used to increase red cells and plasma volume.

10. Packed red blood cells (PRBC) are commonly used to raise Hgb/Hct levels.

11. Platelets are commonly administered to patients with thrombocytopenia.

12. Vital signs are taken immediately prior to giving the blood transfusion and generally every fifteen minutes for one hour and than every half hour for the remainder of the transfusion. However, it is important to follow the healthcare agencies guidelines when administering a blood transfusion.

13. The nurse assesses for fever, chills, tachycardia, tachypnea, dyspnea, hives, skin rash, flushing, gastrointestinal symptoms, hypotension, wheezing, chest pain, headache, and muscle pain.

14. The presence of a fever can indicate an acute hemolytic reaction, febrile non-hemolytic reaction and bacterial sepsis.

15. The presence of tachycardia, tacypnea and dyspnea can indicate acute hemolytic reaction or circulatory overload.

16. The presence of hives and or skin rash can indicate an allergic reaction or anaphylaxis.

17. The presence of flushing can also indicate an acute hemolytic reaction or a febrile non hemolytic reaction.

18. The presence of nausea and or vomiting can indicate an acute hemolytic reaction, anaphylaxis or sepsis.

19. The presences of diarrhea can indicate a graft-versus-host disease or sepsis.

20. The presence of hypotension can indicate an acute hemolytic reaction, anaphylaxis or sepsis.

21. The presence of crackles in the base of the lungs can indicate circulatory overload.

22. If the nurse notices any adverse reactions while administering a blood transfusion, he/she should stop the infusion, infuse the line with normal saline, take vital signs, notify the healthcare provider and the blood bank, obtain blood samples, return the blood and tubing to the blood bank and follow orders according to the healthcare provider.

23. The nurse needs to document the date, time, blood product, patient response and any medication or treatments that were given.

Naso-Gastric and Naso-Enteric Tube Feeding Care

1. NG tube is the abbreviated term for a naso gastric tube.

2. NG tubes are most often used for feedings but can also be used to decompress the stomach.

3. Patients with facial and/or cranial injuries or surgeries should not have NG placement.

4. Yes, the insertion of a feeding tube requires a healthcare provider's order.

5. No, the nurse cannot delegate the verification of a feeding tube to nursing assistive personnel.

6. Yes, the nurse can delegate the administration of a NG tube feeding to nursing assistive personnel if the agency policy does not prohibit.

7. The risk of aspiration is considered a major risk factor when administering NG tube feedings.

8. The nurse inserts small bore feeding tubes nasally or orally.

9. The nurse takes the NG tube and starts measuring by taking the tip of the tube and placing it at the tip of the patient's nose then extending it to the patient's ear lobe and then measure from the earlobe to the patient's xyphoid process and marking this point with a piece of tape.

10. The recommended patient positioning for NG tube insertion is high fowler's position if it is not contraindicated.

11. The initial recommended way to verify if a NG tube is placed properly is through x-ray.

12. The nurse assesses verification prior to using the NG tube for feedings at least every four to six hours and according to the healthcare agency policy.

13. If the patient starts to cough, choke and show signs of altered respiratory status the nurse should stop the insertion of the NG tube immediately.

14. Vomiting, retching, coughing and nasotracheal suctioning can increase the patient's risk for both dislodging the NG tube and aspiration.

15. A gastric feeding tube such as a gastrostomy tube can be inserted if a patient cannot tolerate a small bore feeding tube or requires long term tube feedings.

16. Depending on the type of gastrostomy tube, a physician inserts the tube in one of the following settings: operating room, endoscopy or in radiology.

17. A jejunostomy tube is the feeding tube that is inserted in the jejunum.

18. No, the nurse cannot delegate care of a gastrostomy or jejunostomy tube to nursing assistive personnel.

19. 8 hours is the general amount of time that formula in a tube feeding can hang up for in an open system.

20. 24 hours is the general amount of time that formula in a tube feeding can hang up for in a closed system.

Care of Urinary Catheters

1. Yes, the nurse needs an order to inset a urinary catheter.

2. No, the insertion of a straight or indwelling catheter cannot be delegated to nursing assistive personnel.

3. Yes, the task of routine urinary catheter care and the removal of a urinary catheter can be delegated to nursing assistive personnel.

4. The nurse should document the size and type of the urinary catheter, the patient's response, and specimens obtained as well as the color, odor, consistency, amount and frequency (COCAF) of the urine output.

5. The nurse inserts the urinary catheter into the urethra.

6. After inserting the urinary catheter into the urethra it is than advanced into the urinary bladder.

7. The nurse can leave one catheter in the vagina in order to better visualize placing a new catheter into the urethra.

8. When inserting a urinary catheter in a male patient and there is noted resistance the nurse can instruct the patient to take deep slow breaths to help him relax.

9. If when inserting urinary catheter in a male patient and there is continued resistance even after having the patient do relaxation techniques, the nurse should notify the healthcare provider.

10. A straight or intermittent catheter is used to intermittently remove urine from the bladder, take a sterile urine sample or check for residual urine in the patient's bladder.

11. A foley or indwelling catheter is used for short or long term use and is attached to a closed drainage system.

12. The separate lumen attached to the foley catheter is used to inflate the balloon and keep the catheter in place.

13. If when inflating the balloon on the foley catheter causes the patient to experience pain, the nurse should stop inflating; allow fluid to drain back into the syringe and than attempt to advance the catheter slowly into the urinary bladder.

14. A foley or an indwelling catheter may be inserted for patients with certain wounds, urinary obstruction, post-operatively and to measure urine output.

15. The nurse should note the color, odor, consistency, amount and frequency (COCAF) of the urine collected.

16. The patient's urine collection container should be placed below the level of the bladder.

17. Catheters that are 16fr or greater can cause damage to the urethra and bladder neck and cause bladder spasms.

18. Catheter care provided includes: assessing urine for COCAF, redness and/or discharge at the urethra, signs of burning, pain or discomfort at the catheter site. Catheter care also includes cleansing around the urinary catheter with soap and warm water and following the healthcare facilities policy.

19. When removing an indwelling urinary catheter, the nurse must remove the sterile water from the inflation valve.

20. If the nurse removes sterile water from the inflation valve and feels resistance the nurse should try to remove any sterile water that still remains in the inflation valve.

References

Perry & Potter (2005) clinical Nursing Skills & Techniques 7th edition